Going to the Hospital . . . What Will I See?

And Who Are Those People Wearing Funny Clothes?

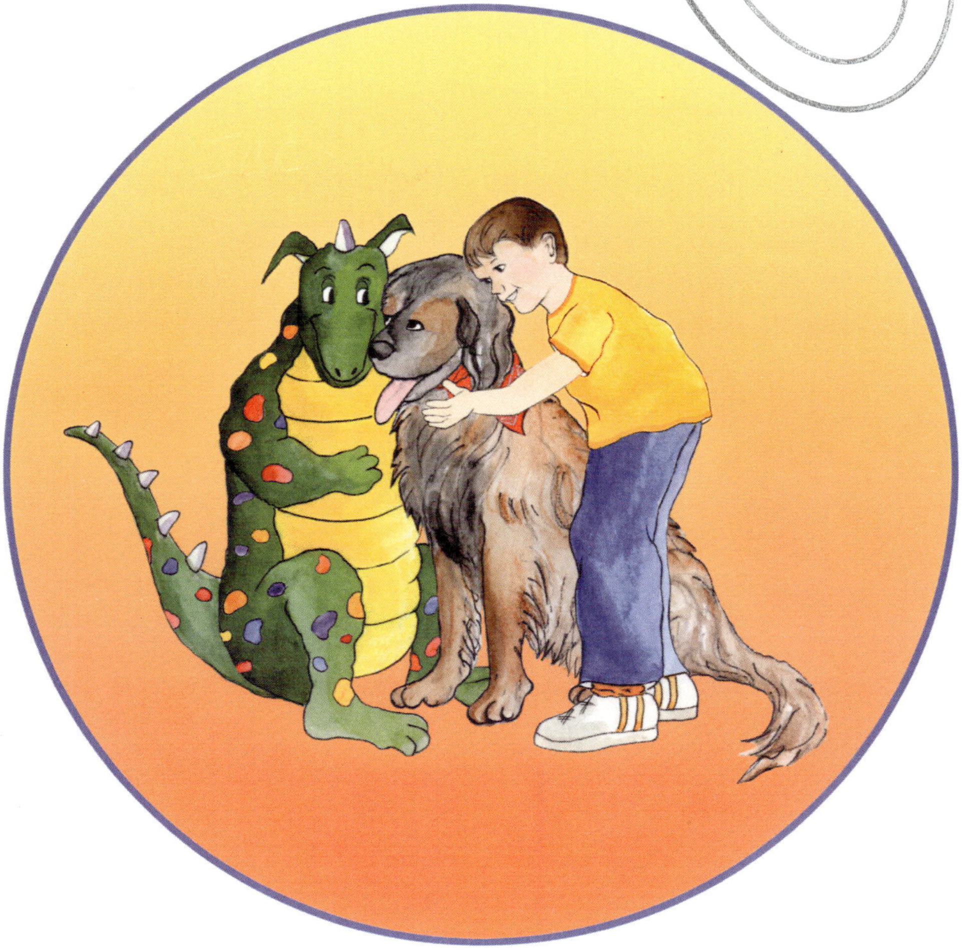

Jaynie R. Wood, M.S., Child Life Specialist
with Jo Berkus
Illustrations by Joan Selwyn

AuthorHouse™
1663 Liberty Drive, Suite 200
Bloomington, IN 47403
www.authorhouse.com
Phone: 1-800-839-8640

First published by AuthorHouse 4/14/2009

ISBN: 978-1-4389-3862-2 (sc)

Library of Congress Control Number: 2008911629

Printed in the United States of America
Bloomington, Indiana

This book is printed on acid-free paper.

This book is dedicated to all Pet Assisted Therapy Dogs, especially **Rowan**, and their handlers who brighten the lives of hospitalized children and their families.

authorHOUSE®

INTRODUCTION:

Going to the Hospital . . . What Will I See? is a book about a journey. The journey will be different for everyone, but the people you meet and the things you see will be very similar. All the people and the special equipment are here to help you feel better.

We begin our journey by walking through the front doors of the hospital. The doors may look very big to you, and this may be your first time going to a hospital. There will be new things to see, new smells, and new feelings. It is our hope that this book will answer many of your questions about your stay in the hospital.

Our patient's name is Kirk. He is coming to the hospital for the first time. Kirk is carrying a stuffed dragon, his favorite toy.

Kirk looks up at his Mom and asks, "Why am I going to the hospital? What will I see?"

And so our story begins . . . .

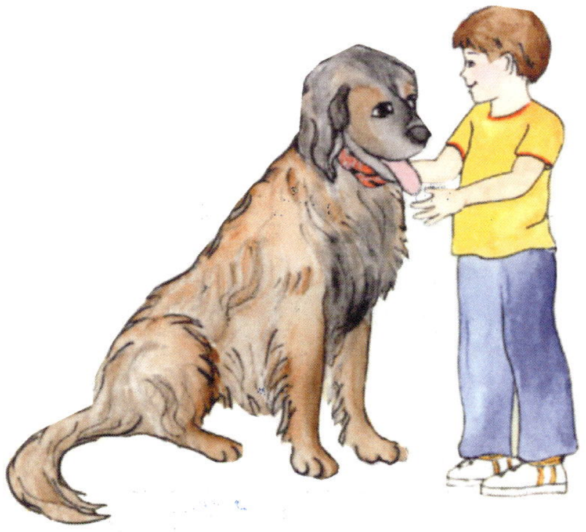

As Kirk and his parents come through the big hospital doors, they are greeted by a woman named Glenda who works in Pediatrics, the special place in the hospital just for children. Glenda is a Child Life Specialist (CLS). A Child Life Specialist is a person who will answer any questions you might have and is someone who will be your friend while you are in the hospital.

"Good morning, you must be Kirk." Kirk nods his head "yes."

"My name is Glenda. Let's take an elevator ride and I will tell you all about this very special place."

Kirk asks, "Where are we going? What will I see?"

Glenda replies, "The elevator will take us to the Pediatrics floor, a special place in the hospital just for children. You will see doctors, nurses and many people who work in the hospital. All these people are here to help you feel better. You will also see other boys and girls who are staying in the hospital just like you."

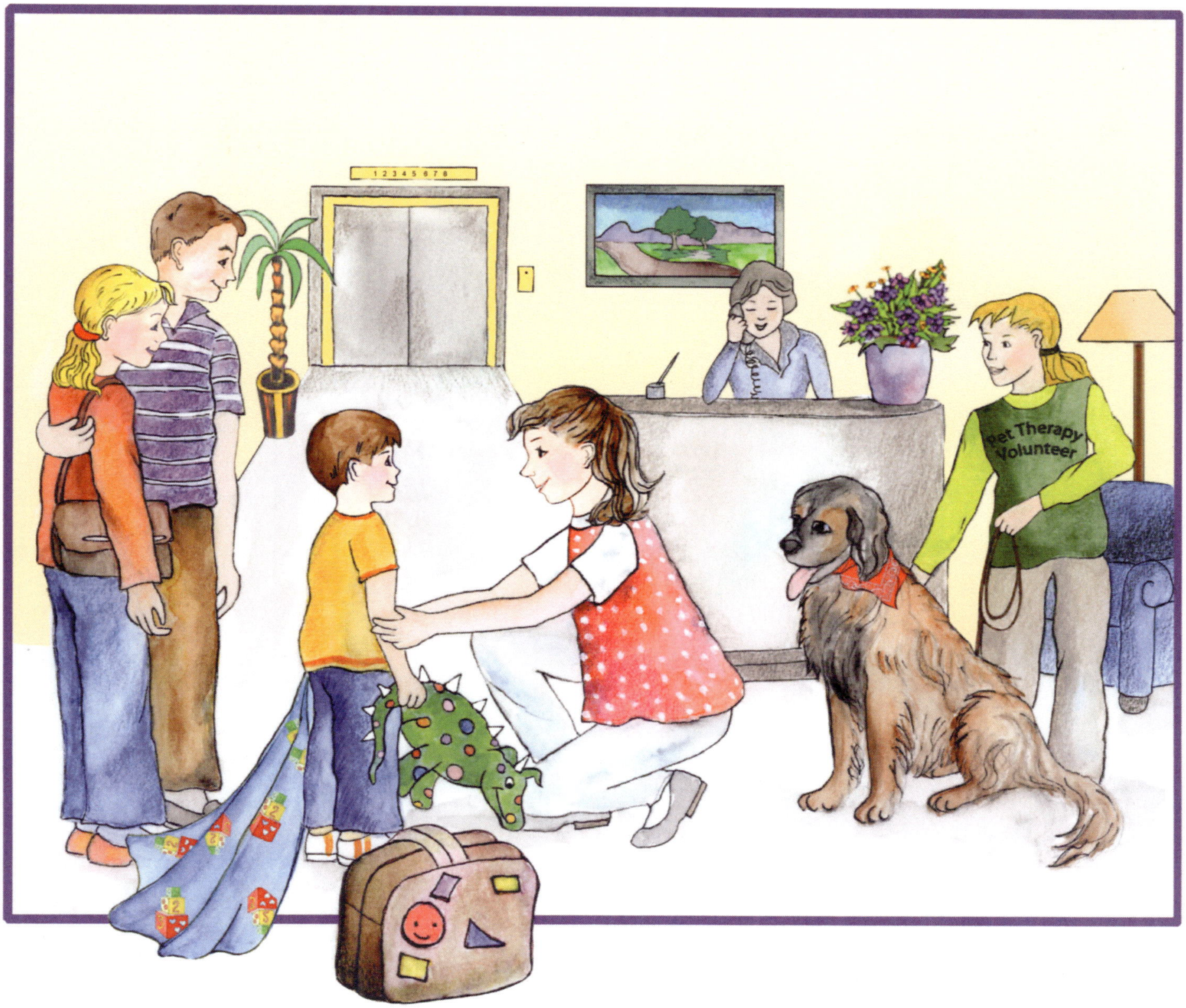
Pet Therapy
Volunteer

As the elevator door opens, POOF, something magical happens. Kirk's favorite stuffed dragon is walking beside him.

"What happened to you," Kirk asks. And the dragon responds, "I thought I would come with you on your hospital journey, but you are the only one who can see me. That is our secret."

"Cool," says Kirk, delighted at his wonderful surprise.

Kirk, the dragon and his parents walk down the hall to Pediatrics where Nurse Bobbi greets them as they arrive. Suddenly Kirk spies a huge wagging tail sticking out of one of the doorways, and he thinks 'this may not be such a bad place after all.'

Can you find the wagging tail?

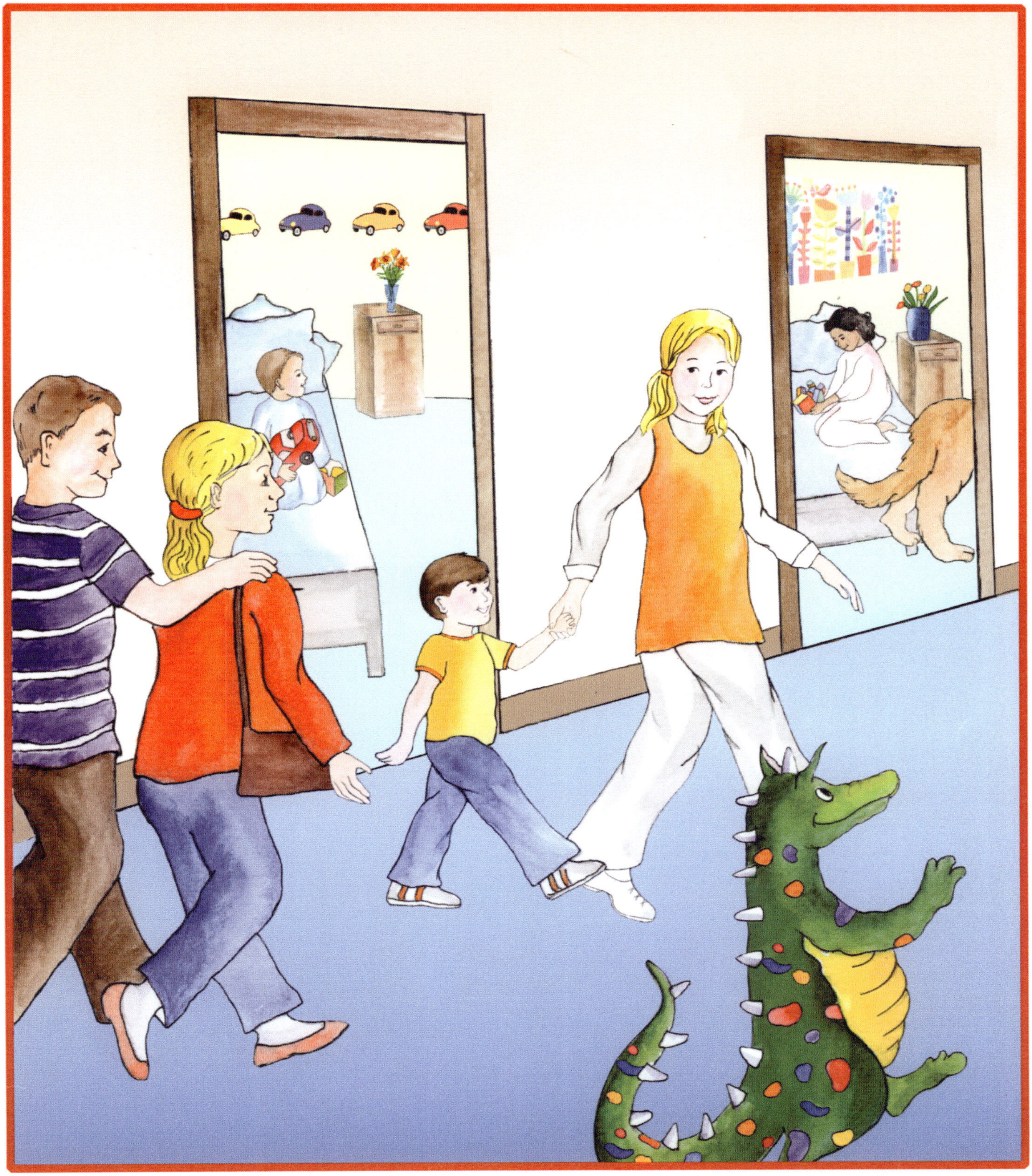

Nurse Bobbi says, "I will be your nurse while you stay with us. Let's start by measuring your height, weight and vital signs."

Kirk asks, "What are vital signs?"

"That is a very good question. Vital signs are your temperature, your blood pressure and your heart rate. Since everyone is different, we need to know how your body works so we can help you feel better."

Kirk asks, "Will it hurt?"

Nurse Bobbi leans down and says, "No, it will not hurt. I will explain everything I do and will let you know if something will be uncomfortable." Kirk sighs and sits down.

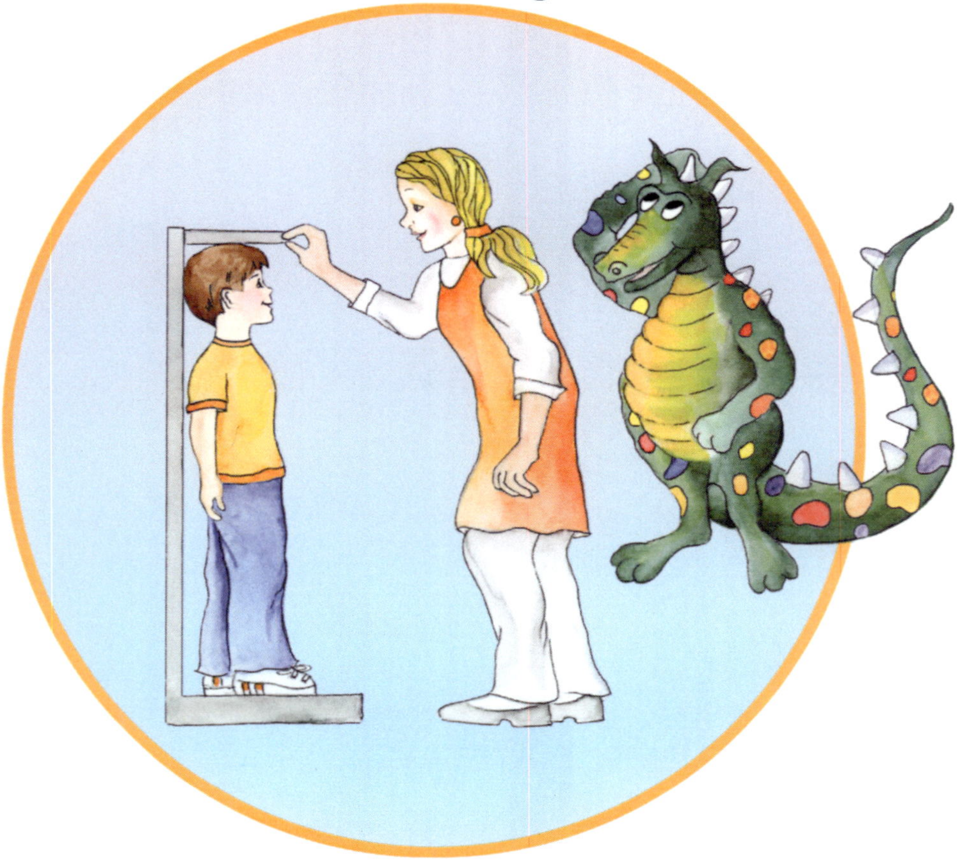

"Let's begin with the blood pressure cuff. The cuff feels soft and will give your arm a little hug. It tells me how your blood is moving throughout your body. Next I will gently roll a thermometer across your forehead and down the side of your cheek. It might feel a little tickly but it won't hurt."

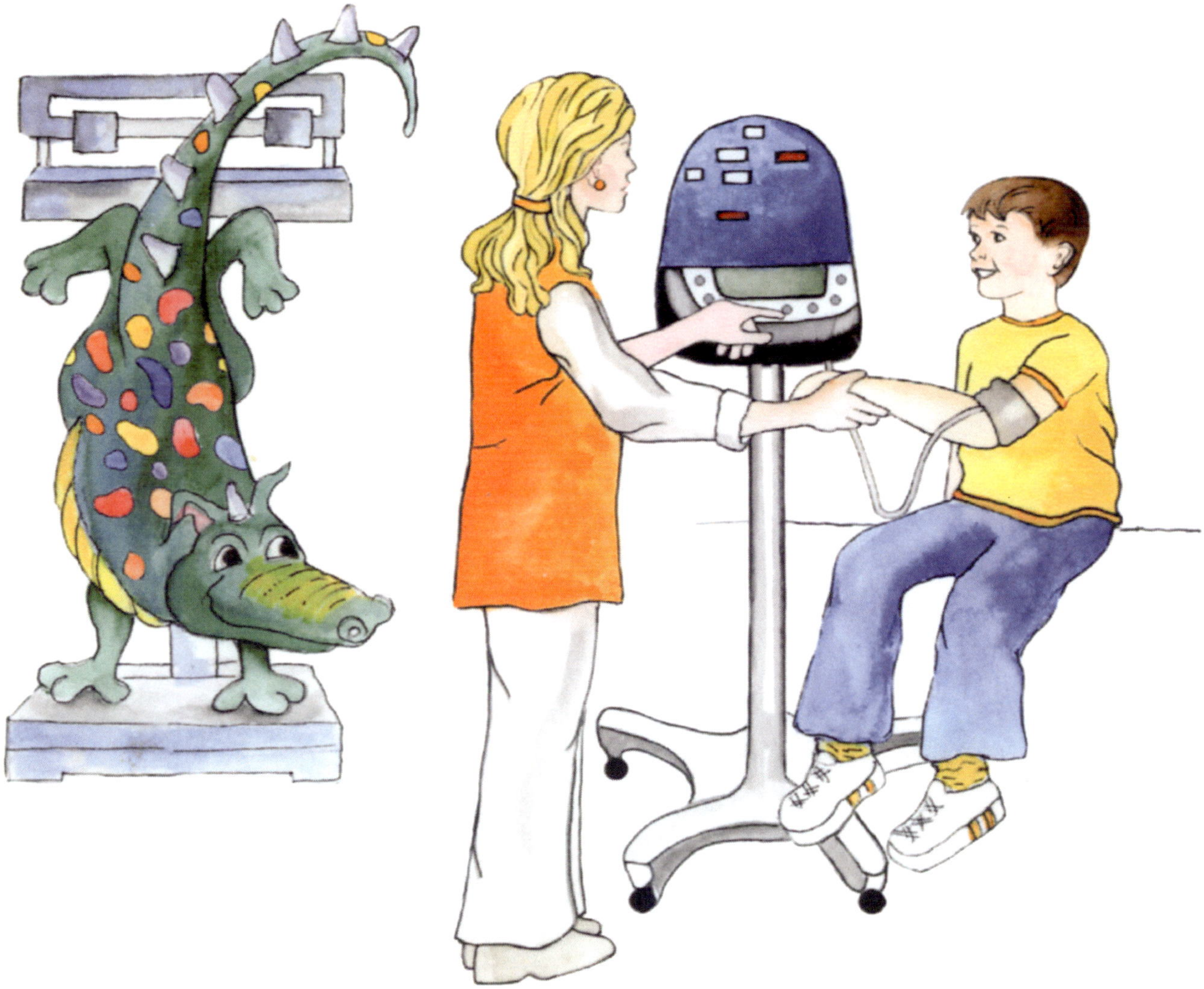

As they finish up, Glenda comes into the room holding a stuffed dog, a gift from the hospital. She tells him the dog can go into the operating room with him. Kirk thinks it looks just like the dog he saw when he first entered the hospital.

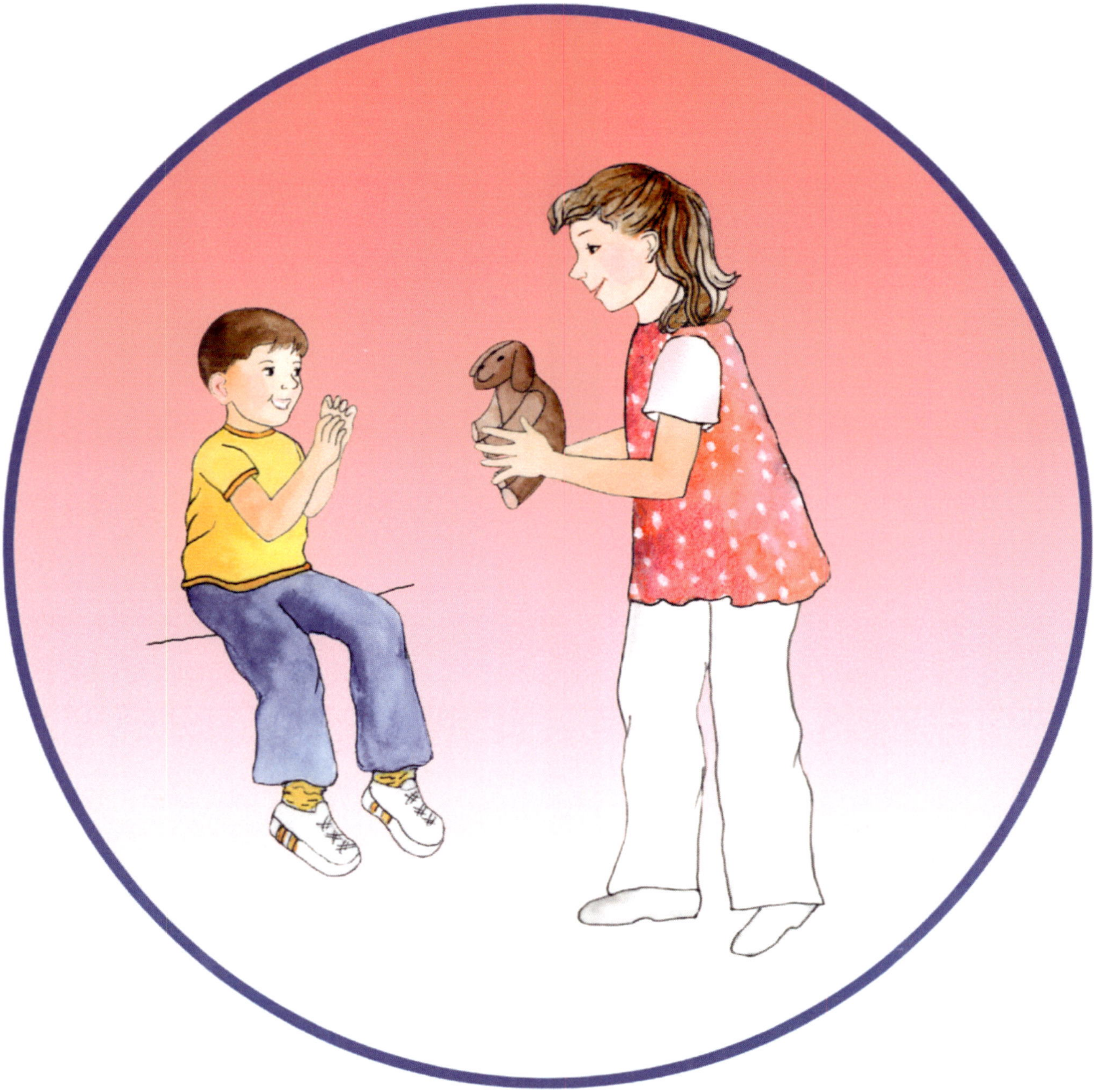

Next Nurse Bobbi puts a special cream on Kirk's skin, telling him it will make his skin feel a little tingly. It will help to start his I.V.

Kirk looks sad and asks, "What is an I.V.? Will it hurt?"

Bobbie reaches over and takes Kirk's hand. "Some patients say they feel a slight poke and some say they don't feel anything at all. That's why we use the special cream, so we can find the best place to send good medicine to your body. I will gently tap your arm so the veins will look bigger. When they get bigger, it is easier for us to see them. Watch as I tap your vein."

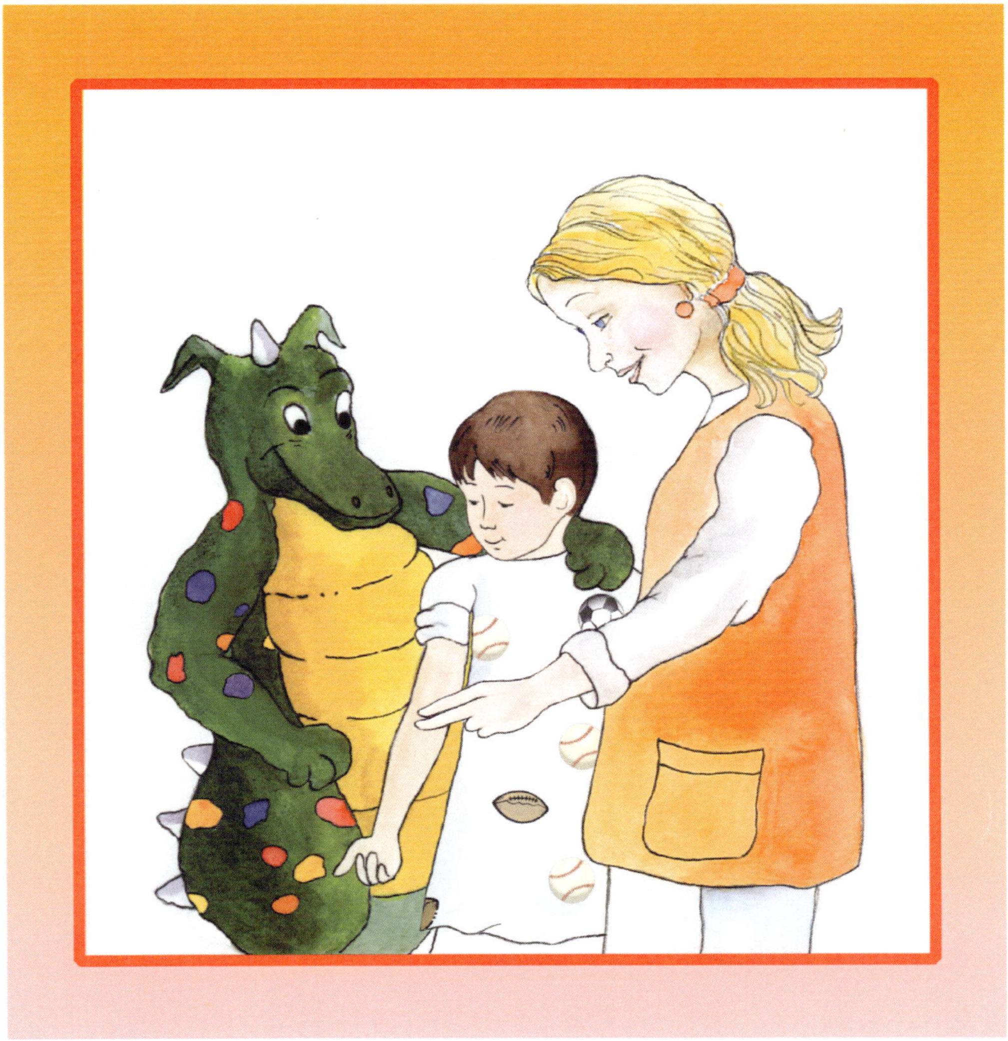

"Next I will put a tourniquet on your arm. It is like a big squishy rubber band and it will give your arm a soft squeeze. I will take a good look at your veins, chose a vein that looks just right and start your I.V. If you hold very still, it will help me get the I.V. started more quickly."

Glenda comes into the room and tells Kirk, "It also helps if you take slow deep breaths. This makes the veins look bigger. You can use your other hand to hold on to your Mom or Dad, or you can hold my hand. You can squeeze our hands as hard as you can and it won't hurt us."

"Then Nurse Bobbi will take a very tiny tube (we call it a Catheter) and slide it into your vein. By using the special cream, almost all of our patients say the tube is in before they know it."

Kirk still feels a little scared, but he says that he is ready to have his I.V. started. Kirk and his Mom follow Nurse Bobbi to the treatment room. It takes just a few minutes and soon they are back in Kirk's room.

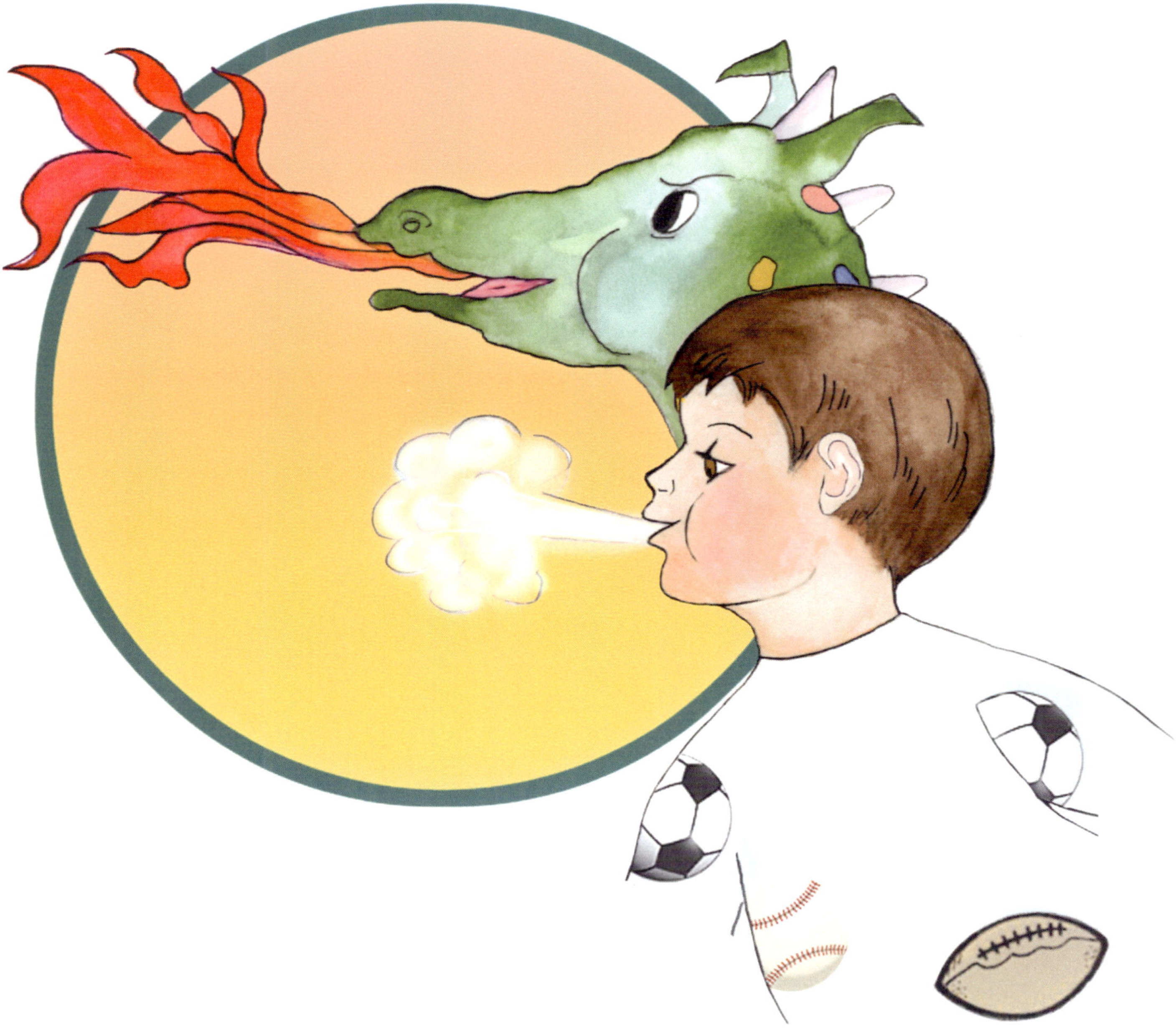

Later Nurse Bobbi stops by with a special hospital bracelet in her hand, which she fastens on Kirk's wrist.

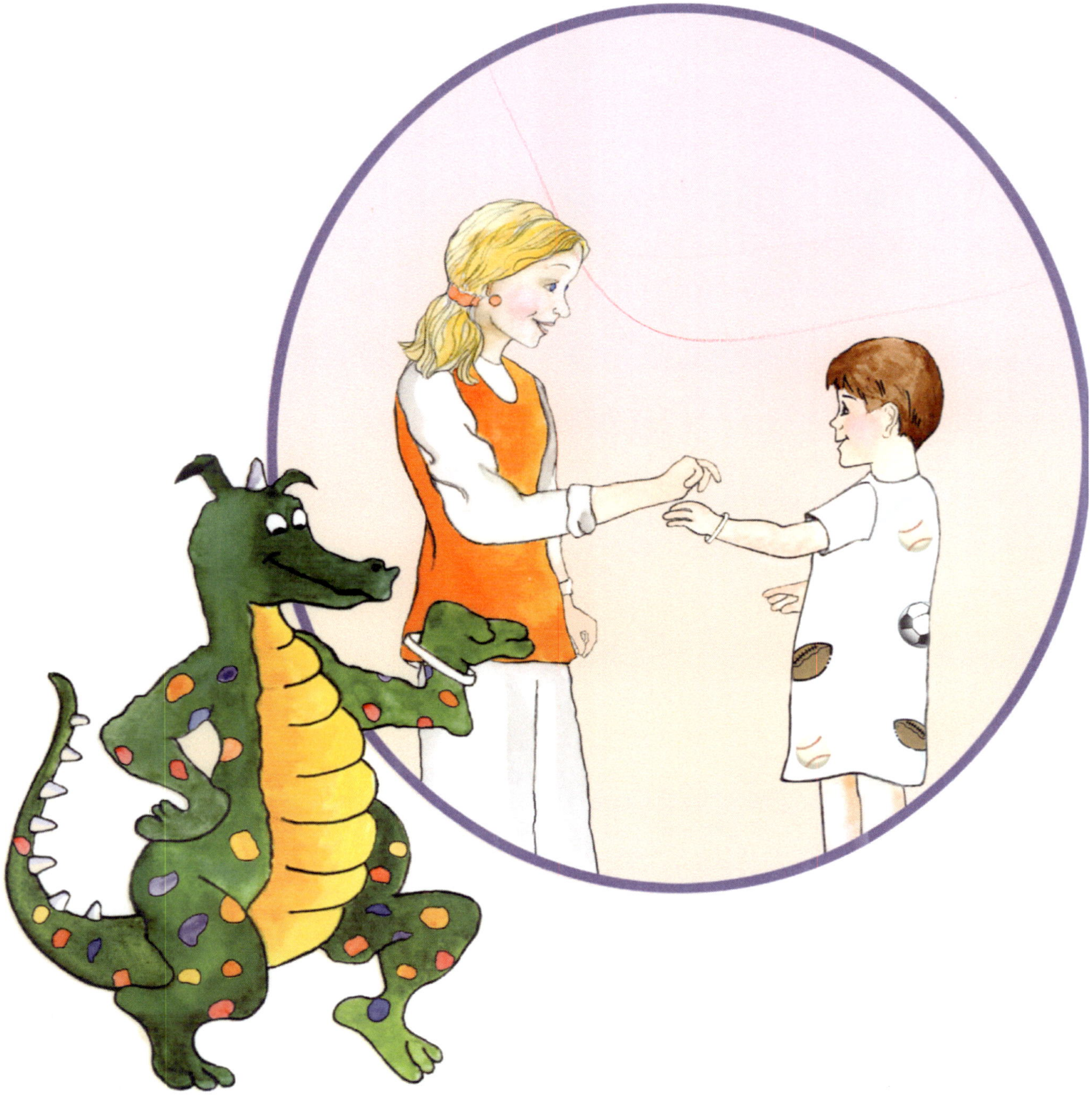

Shortly afterwards, a gurney with big blue wheels rolls smoothly into Kirk's room. Kirk thinks it looks a little like his bed at home, except this one has wheels.

Glenda tells Kirk, "When you are ready to go to the operating room, you will climb onto the gurney and we will gently roll you down the hallway. The gurney will take you to a place that is similar to the garage where your Dad has his car fixed. Here in the hospital we call it the Operating Room. In this room the doctors help people like you feel better."

Kirk asks, "Am I going to the operating room?"

"You are," replies Glenda.

"Can my Mom and Dad come with me?"

Glenda says, "Let's get you on the gurney and I will answer all your questions."

"Your first stop will be in the Pre-Surgical room which is down the hall. Your Mom and Dad will be with you. It will give you a chance to meet some of the people who will be with you in the operating room."

Kirk says, "I'm still scared."

Glenda tells him "It's OK to be scared, but all the people are here to help you feel better. There will always be someone with you. Let me tell you what each of these people do."

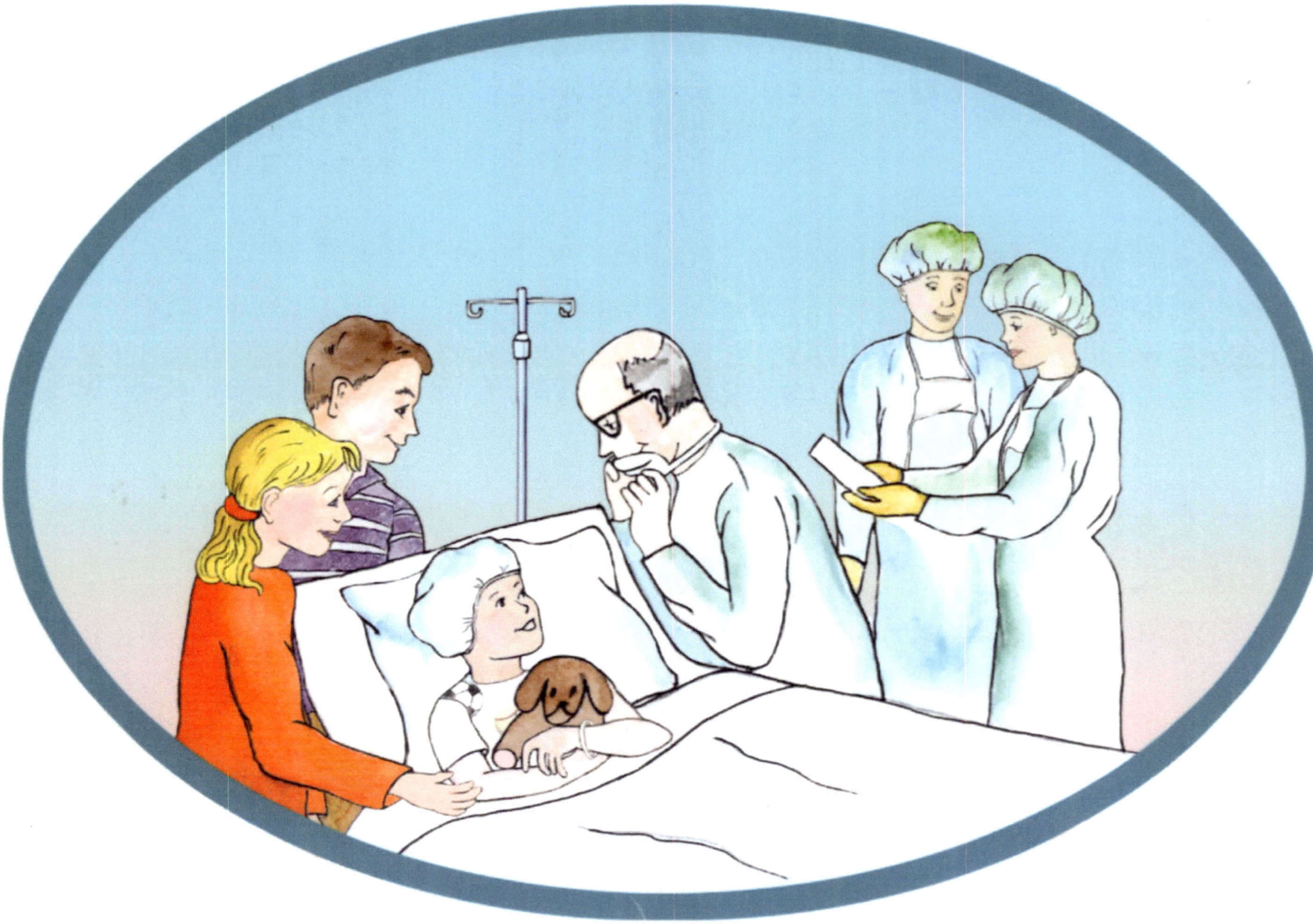

"One of the doctors is called a surgeon, a doctor in charge of helping you feel better. The second doctor is an Anesthesiologist. Because that is a difficult word to say, we call him the Sleepy Doctor. He will make sure that you sleep peacefully during the time you are in the operating room. The third person is a nurse who helps the doctors. In no time at all, you will be awake."

"Are you sure I will wake up?" asks Kirk who starts to cry.

"Yes, I am sure of that. The sleepy doctor has a very important job. The sleepy doctor gives you special medicine through the little tube in your vein. You will take a nice nap while you are in the room. When the surgeon is finished, the sleepy doctor will stop giving you the special sleepy medicine and you will wake up and see your Mom and Dad."

After all their questions are answered, Mom and Dad give Kirk a big hug and tell him they will be right next to him when he wakes up. Then Kirk takes a short ride into the Operating Room that has been prepared just for him.

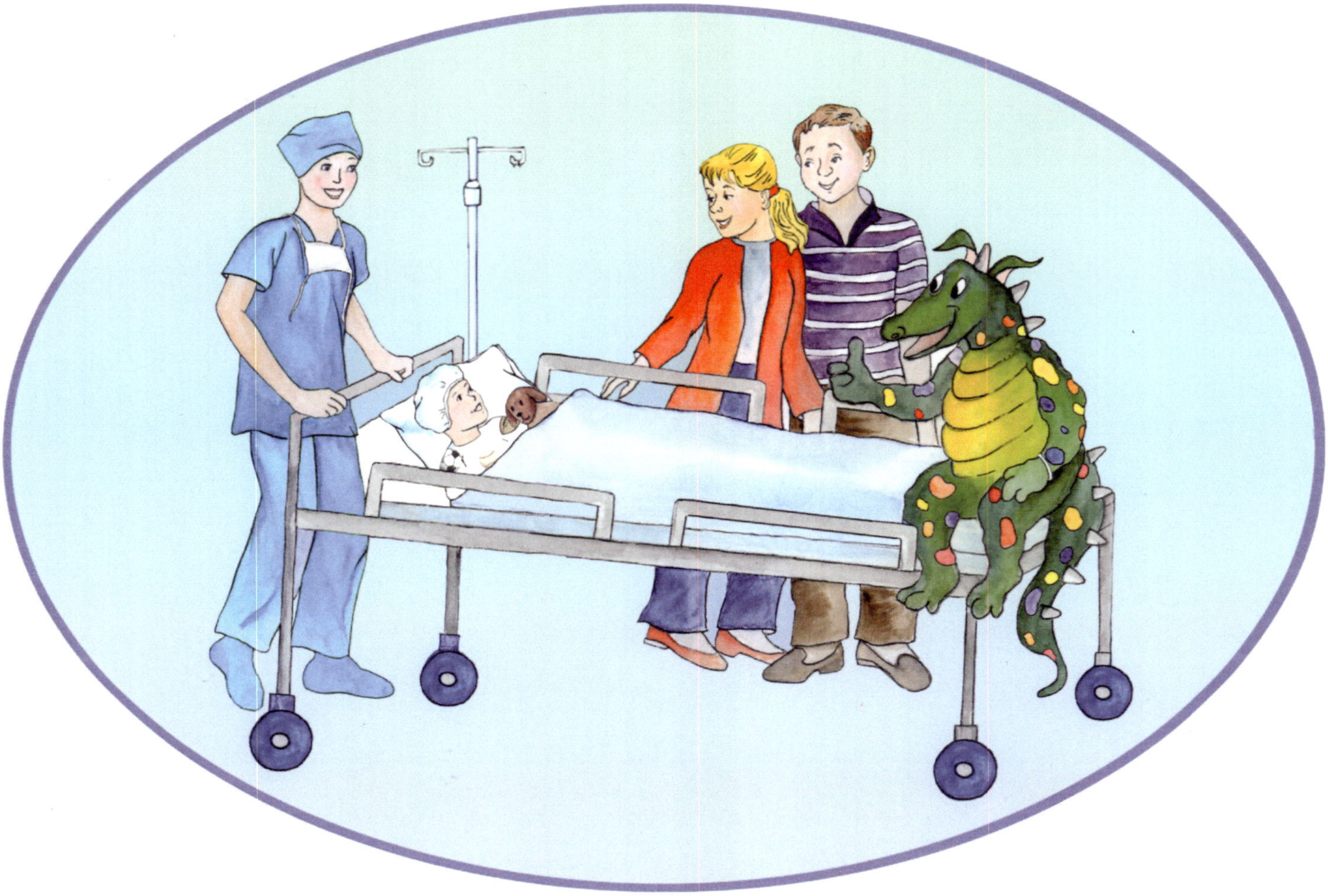

Everyone in the room is wearing special clothing. They have funny paper hats on their heads and paper covers over their mouths and shoes. It seems to Kirk that it is almost like a party. The room is chilly so the nurse places a warm blanket over Kirk. It feels very good.

Next the nurse puts little sticky pads on Kirk's chest. They are used to send signals to a big machine that will monitor your heartbeat and your blood pressure. She tells Kirk, "You can watch the machine make funny squiggly lines on the screen."

Then she puts a blood pressure cuff on Kirk's arm, but Kirk already knows how that feels and he isn't afraid. The nurse also places a little rubber cover on one of Kirk's fingers. It looks a little bit like a finger puppet.

The nurse explains that it will monitor how much oxygen is in his body. "The doctor needs to know your oxygen level to make sure you are taking nice deep breaths."

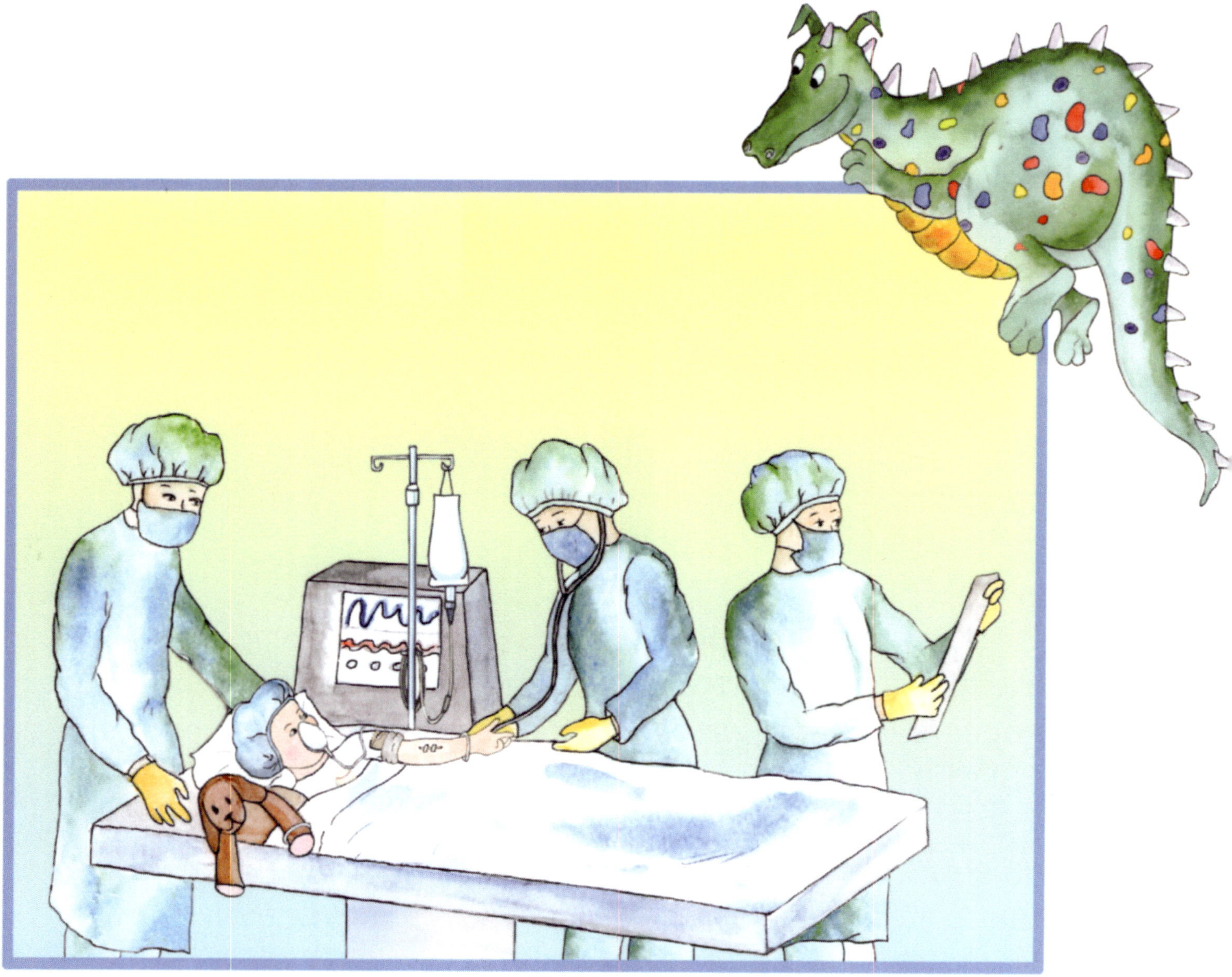

When she is finished, the nurse asks Kirk how he is feeling.

"I'm OK, but I'm still a little scared."

The nurse says, "What are you most scared about?"

Kirk tells her, "Going to sleep."

Then the sleepy doctor leans over and says, "Remember Kirk that is what I do best. I will give you some medicine through the tube in your arm and it will not hurt. When the surgeon is all finished, I just stop giving you the medicine and you will wake up. Your Mom and Dad will be there waiting for you. In fact . . . you might be a little sleepy very soon."

"No, I'm not . . ." and with that, Kirk falls asleep dreaming of eating a huge ice cream cone covered with sprinkles.

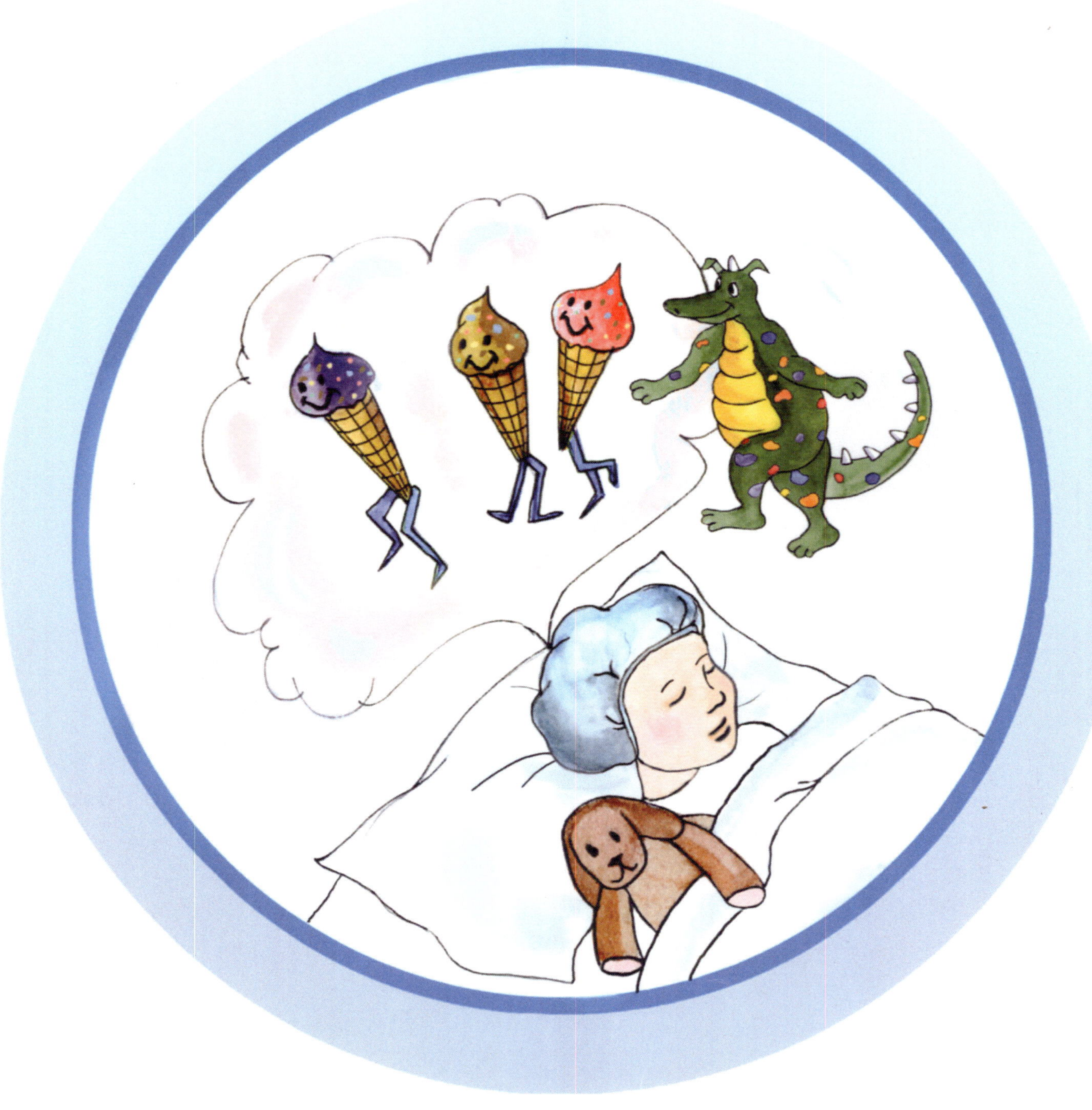

The next thing Kirk remembers is hearing someone call his name. As he wakes up he sees his father come into the room, and he sees his mother right by his side, just as promised.

Kirk's mother says, "We're all finished Sweetheart. How do you feel?"

"My tummy feels funny and I'm thirsty," says Kirk.

As Nurse Bobbi comes by to check on Kirk, she tells him she will bring some medicine to help his tummy feel better. As soon as Kirk gets the medicine, he takes a nap.

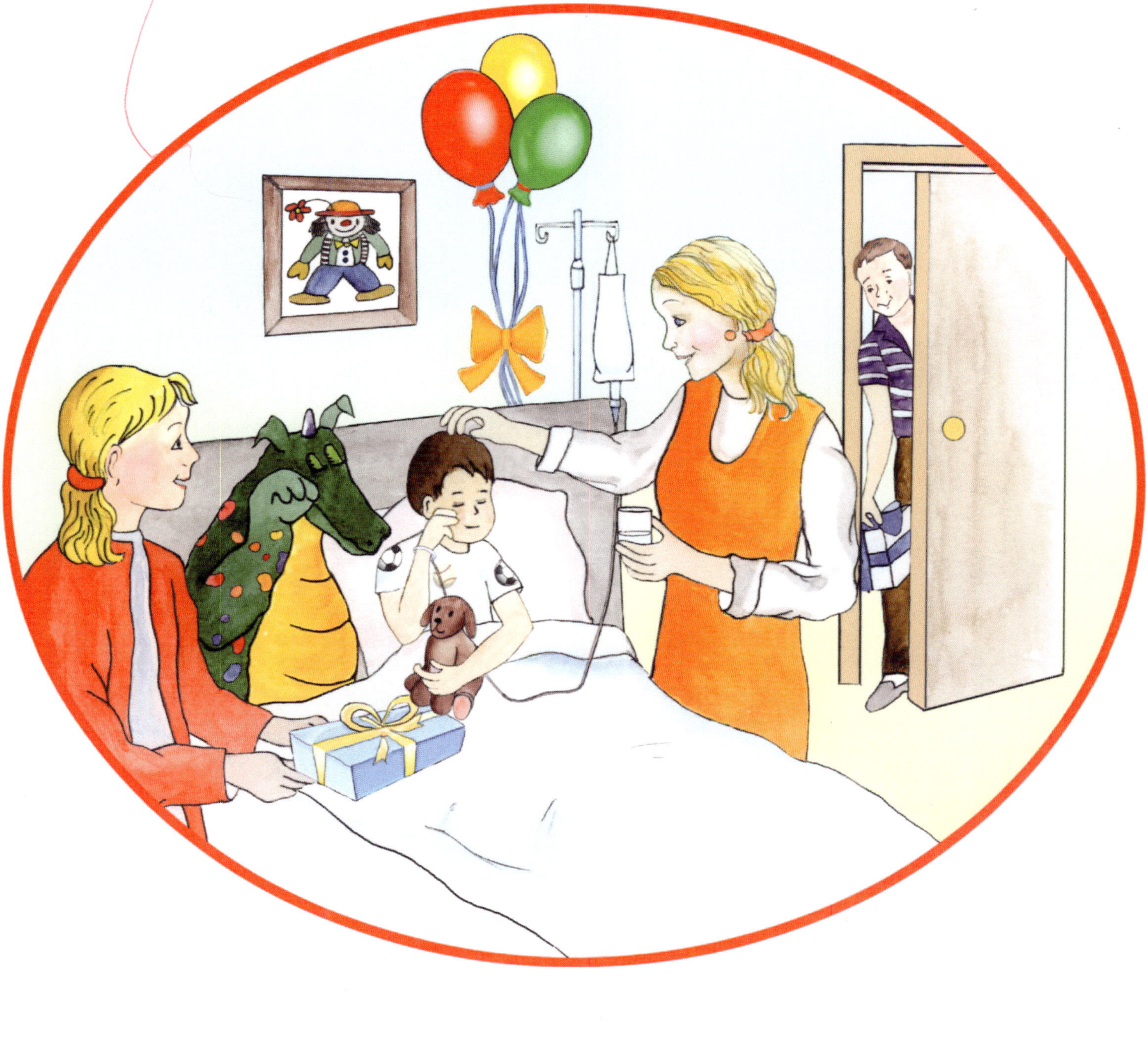

When he wakes up, Nurse Bobbi comes in and asks, "How are you feeling Kirk?"

"My tummy hurts and I'm REALLY thirsty."

"Well, we will take care of that in just a minute. First I need to find out just how bad your tummy feels. I have a chart that will help us. If your tummy does not hurt at all, it is a "0." If you have a very bad tummy ache, it will be a "10." Can you tell me what your tummy feels like?" Kirk thinks it's about a "6."

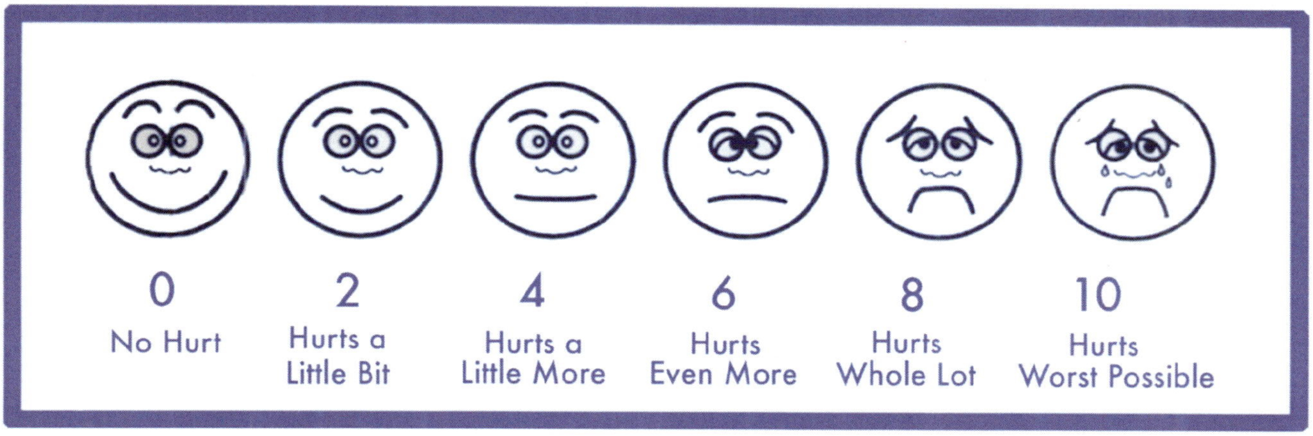

Next Nurse Bobbi asks him to point to the spot where his tummy hurts the most. Then she tells Kirk she will be right back with his medicine and some cold juice to drink.

After Kirk takes his medicine and drinks some of his juice, he drifts off to sleep for the night. His Mom settles into the sleeper chair near Kirk's bed and Kirk's father goes home.

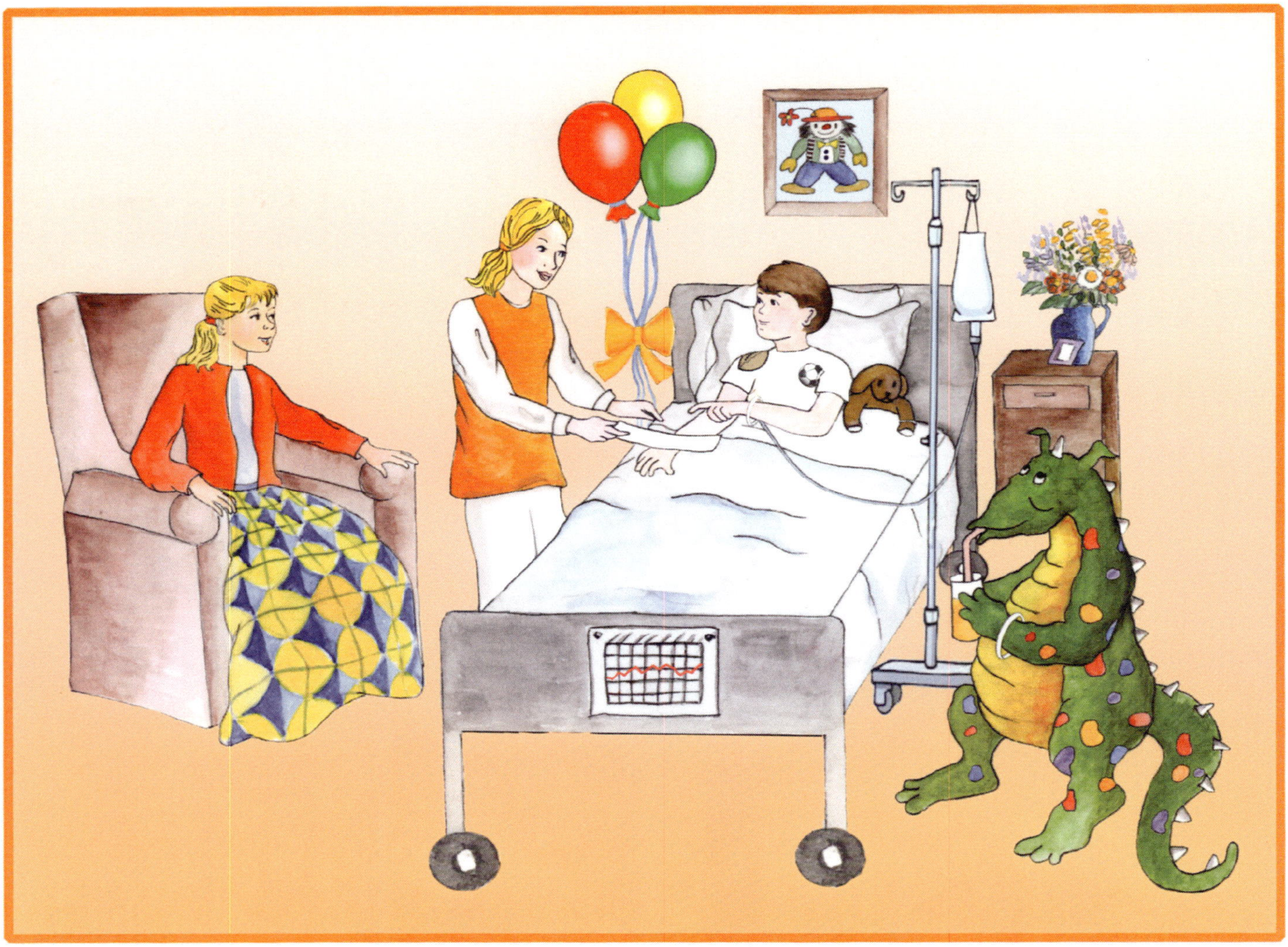

The following morning, Kirk wakes up bright and early. He feels better and he is very hungry. A few minutes later Nurse Bobbi comes in with a breakfast tray and tells Kirk the surgeon will soon be stopping by to see him. As Kirk and his Mom finish breakfast, the doctor comes into the room.

"Good morning Kirk, you look like you are feeling better."

"My tummy doesn't hurt as much as it did last night," says Kirk.

"I'm glad to hear that. I need to listen to your heart and lungs, and I'd like to listen to your tummy too," says the surgeon.

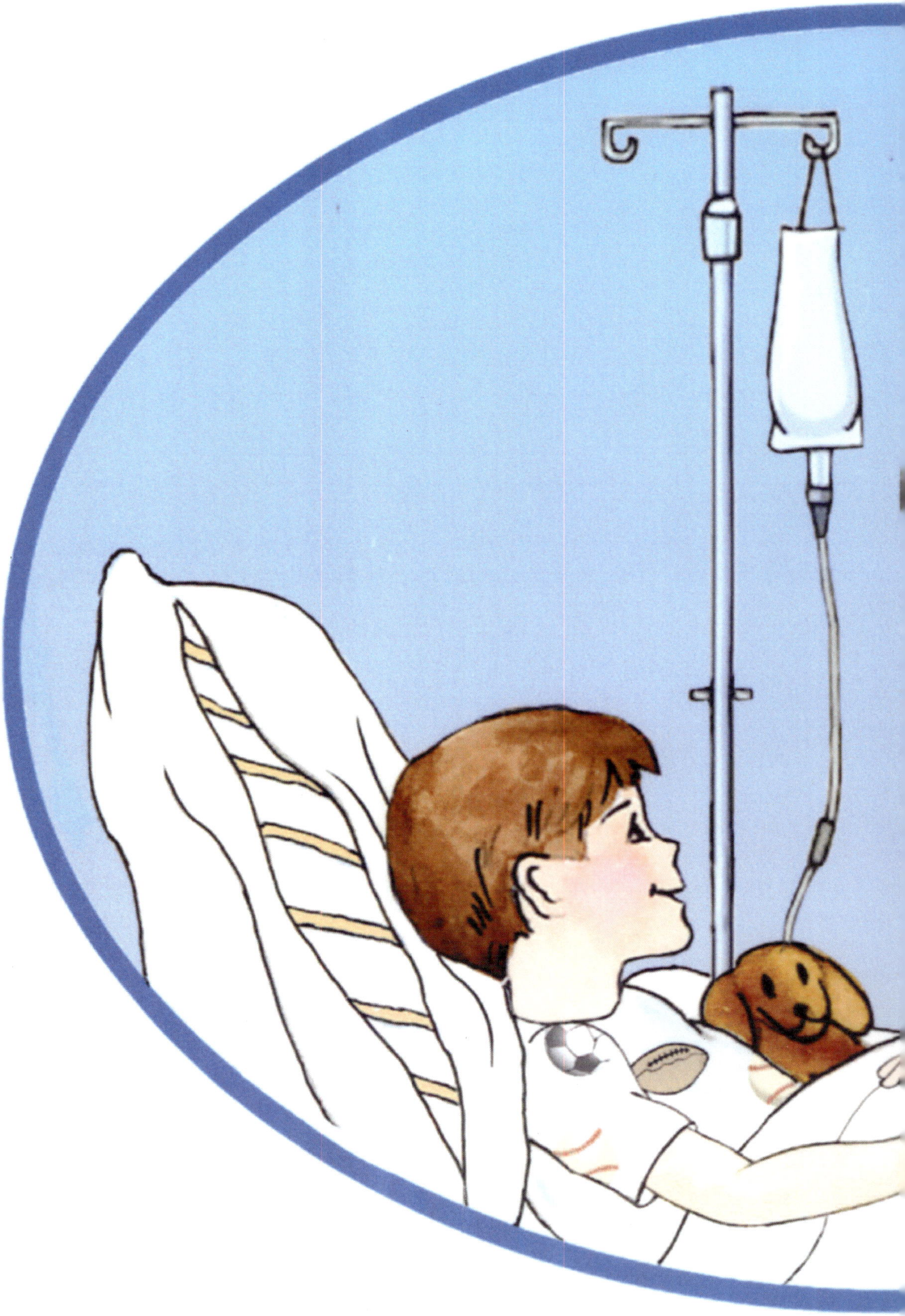

"How do you listen to my tummy?" Kirk asks.

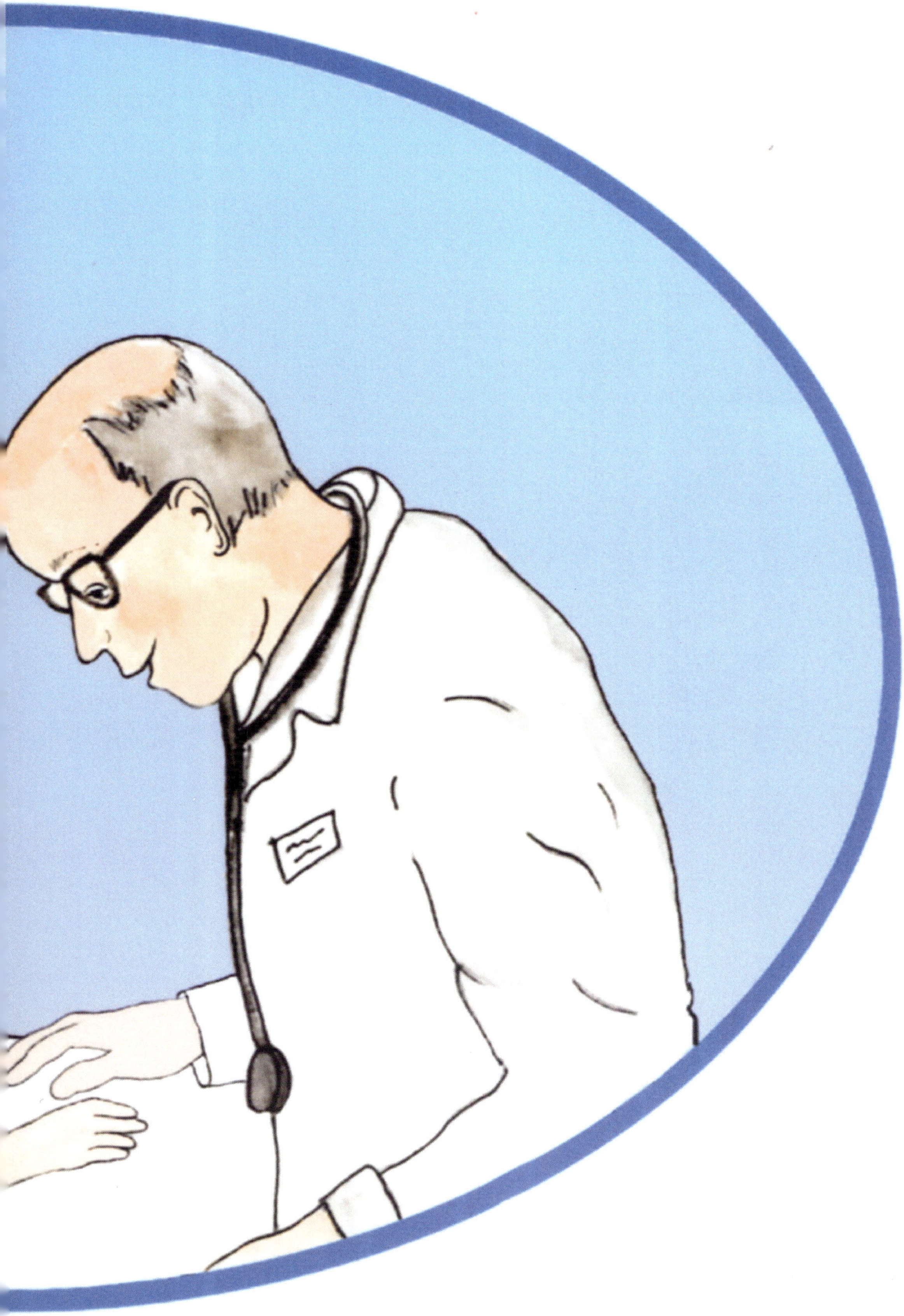

"With a stethoscope, just like I listened to your heart and lungs. It's sort of like ear phones that let you listen to music, only I'm listening to the music of your body."

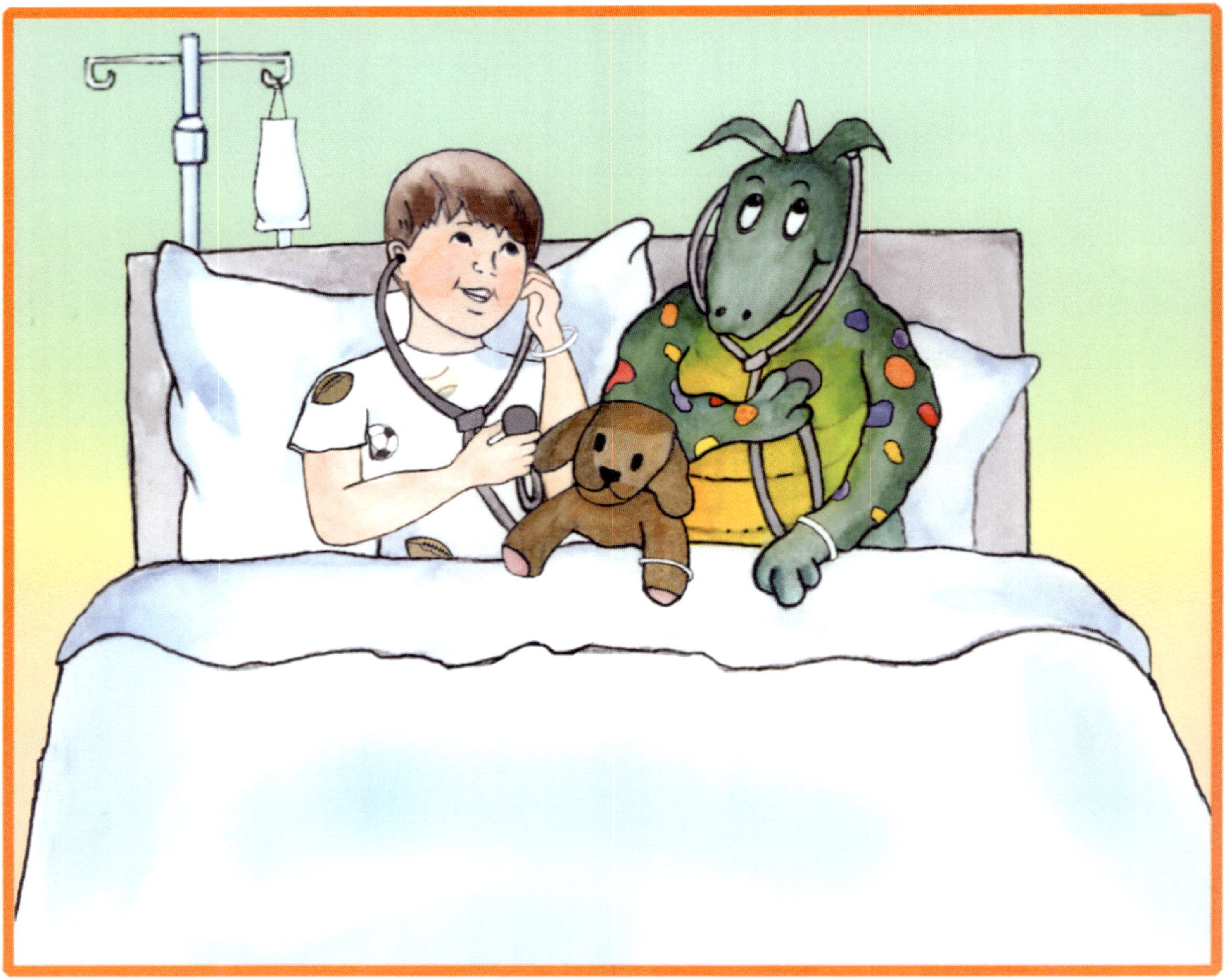

Kirk asks, "What do my heart and lungs say?"

"Listening to your heart tells me everything is working well, and listening to your lungs tells me you are taking nice deep breaths."

And with that, the doctor takes the stethoscope from around his neck and lets Kirk listen to the sounds his body is making.

"Oh," says Kirk. "I can hear it go *thumpa, thumpa, thumpa.* It must mean I'm OK."

The surgeon agrees with him and says, "I'll have you get up and walk around a little bit and by lunch time you should be able to go home." Kirk smiles at the thought of being back in his own house.

Glenda walks into Kirk's room and says. "Good morning Kirk. The doctor says you are doing well this morning. Would you like to go to the playroom?"

"I'm ready," says Kirk. "Can we go right now?"

Glenda tells him she'll return in a few minutes to take him to the playroom.

When she returns, Kirk is sitting on the side of his bed, ready to go to the playroom.

The playroom is filled with books and toys and Kirk decides to stay there for a little while. While he is there, he finds a book to take back to his room.

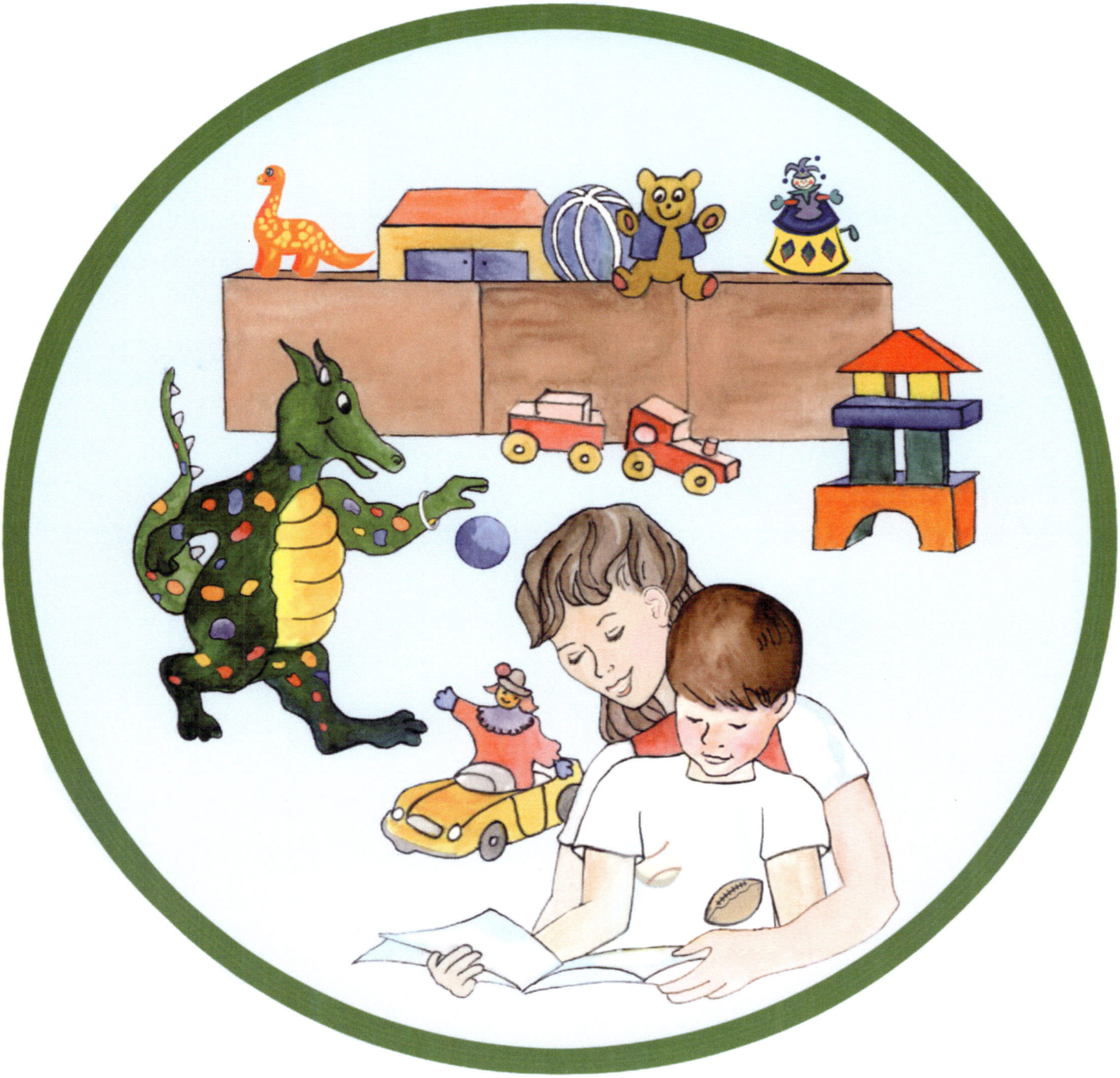

As Kirk and his Mom are reading, Glenda appears in the doorway with a volunteer who is holding onto a dog leash.

She asks, "Would you like a visit from a Therapy dog?"

"Oh yes," exclaims Kirk, and in comes this big teddy bear of a dog named Rowan, who promptly jumps up on Kirk's bed and lies down next to him. Kirk pats the dog's big head and rubs her tummy. Her fur is so soft and silky. Kirk giggles as Rowan lays her head on his pillow and he gives the dog a big hug. They are both very happy.

Just then Nurse Bobbi comes back into the room to take out Kirk's I.V. She gasps and says, "Oh my, where is Kirk? Did he go home without saying good-bye?" Suddenly Kirk's happy face pops up over Rowan's head, his chin resting in the dog's soft fur.

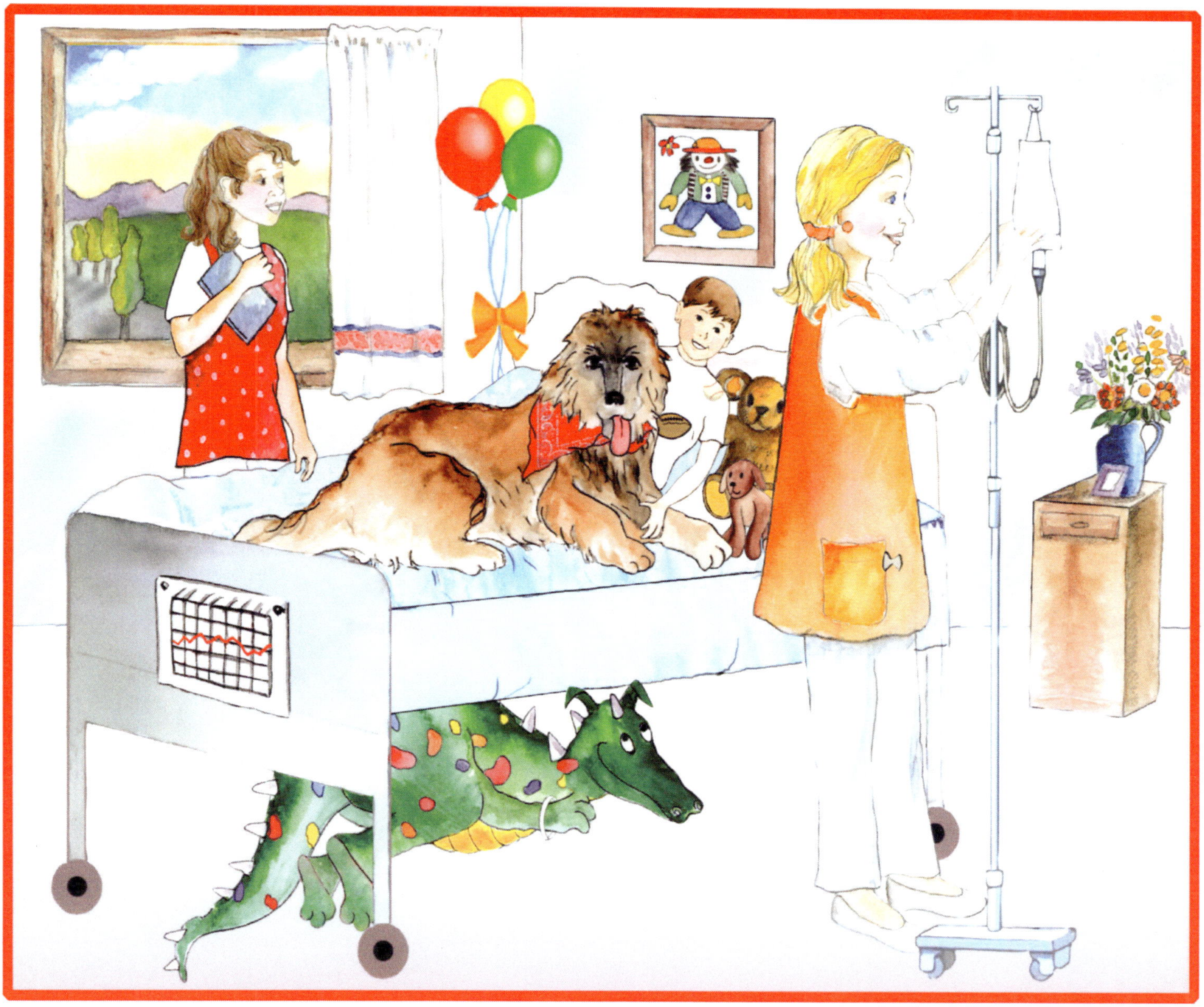

"Since you will be going home today, I can remove your I.V."

Kirk says, "How do you do that?"

"Taking out the I.V. will not hurt at all. The first thing we do is remove the tape. I have some magic tape remover with me. Do you want to help?" asks Nurse Bobbi.

"I'm not sure. What do I have to do?" asks Kirk.

"Just tear open the package, take out the wipe and start rubbing the tape on your arm," says Nurse Bobbi.

Kirk says, "Wow, this really stinks, but the tape is coming off." Kirk didn't even notice that the tube in his arm had been removed.

"When will you take out the I.V," asks Kirk.

"It is already out."

"I didn't even feel you take it out," says Kirk.

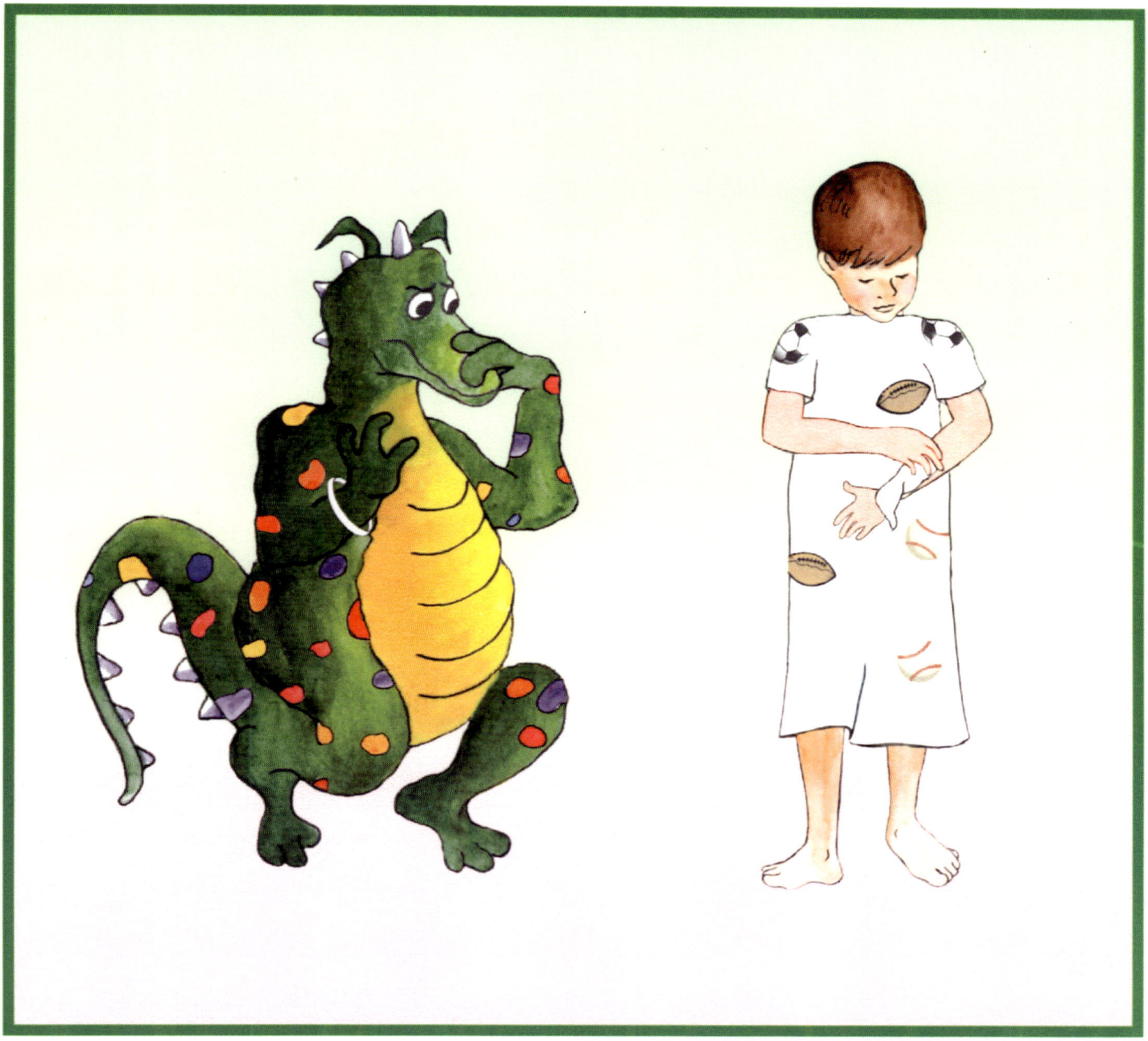

"Well, let's put a band-aid on and then I'll go over the instructions for going home," says Nurse Bobbi. With that, Rowan hops off the bed and heads off to visit the next patient. Nurse Bobbi assures Kirk that Rowan will be back before he leaves.

"Why do I need instructions?" asks Kirk. "My Mommy and Daddy already know how to take care of me."

"Of course they do, but these are special things for your Mom and Dad to know because you just had surgery."

After Nurse Bobbi reviews all the special things for Kirk's Mom and Dad to do when Kirk returns home, she gets him ready to leave the hospital.

"Why do I have to ride in a wheelchair?" asks Kirk.

"Every patient leaving the hospital gets one last ride in the wheel chair. It's kind of our special way to say good-bye to you."

As Kirk travels down the long hallway, Glenda, Nurse Bobbi and all the nice people he met wave good-bye to Kirk. Kirk waves back and thanks all of his friends.

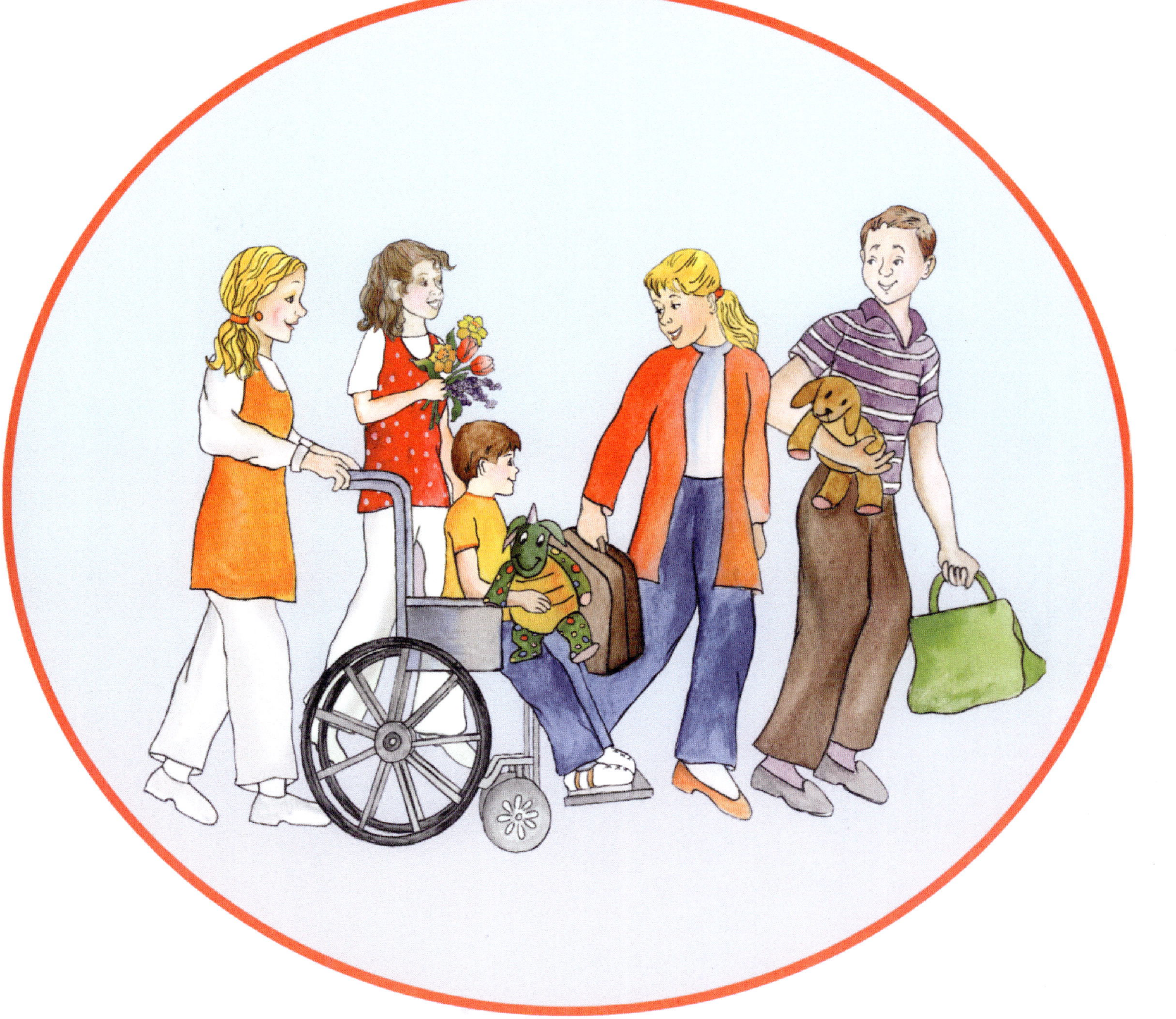

As they reach the elevator, someone is waiting to say good-bye to Kirk. Can you guess who it is?

If you said Rowan, you are so right!

Rowan follows Kirk into the elevator. It is a little crowded, but everyone starts laughing when Rowan's big tail thumps noisily against the elevator wall.

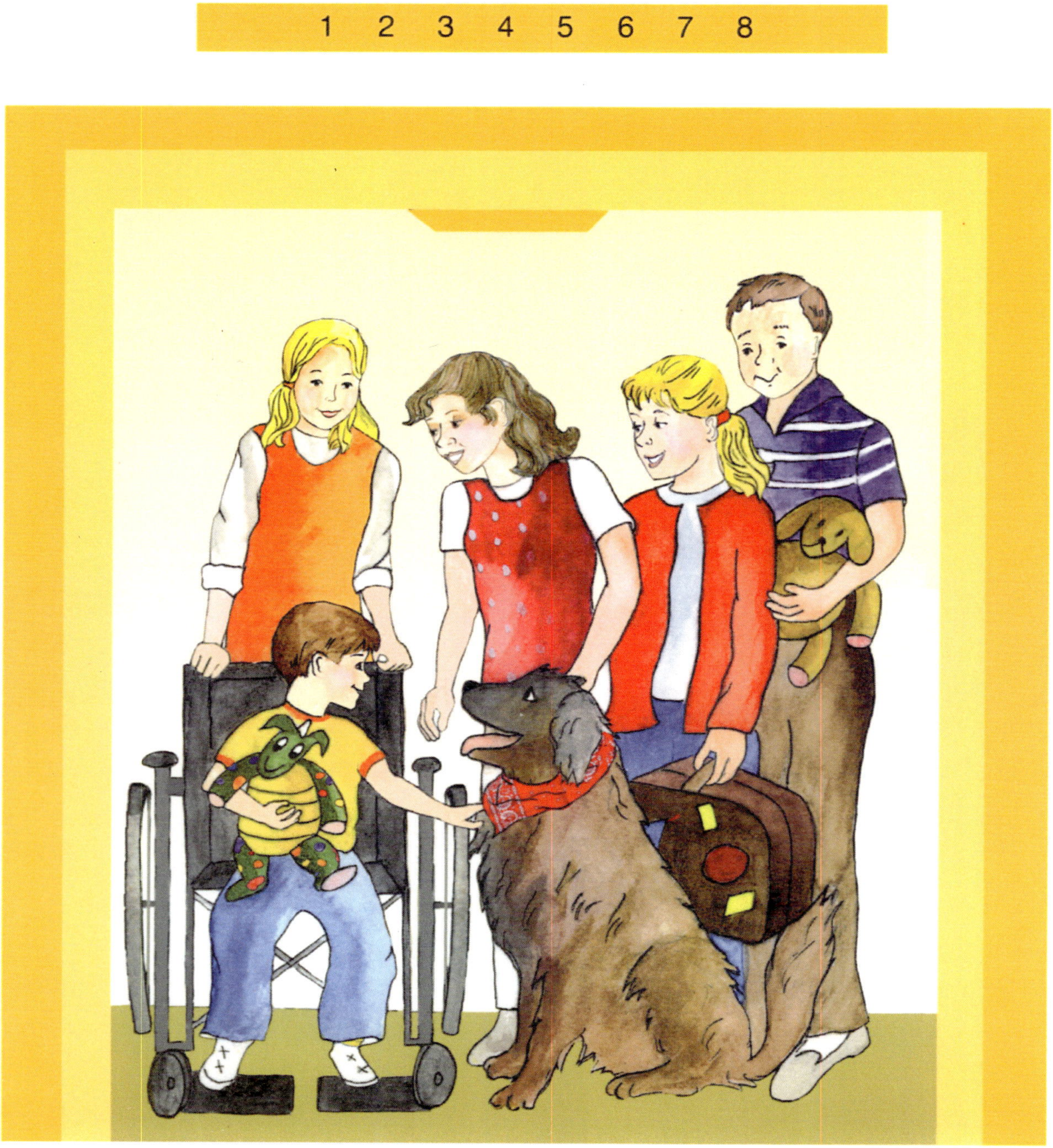

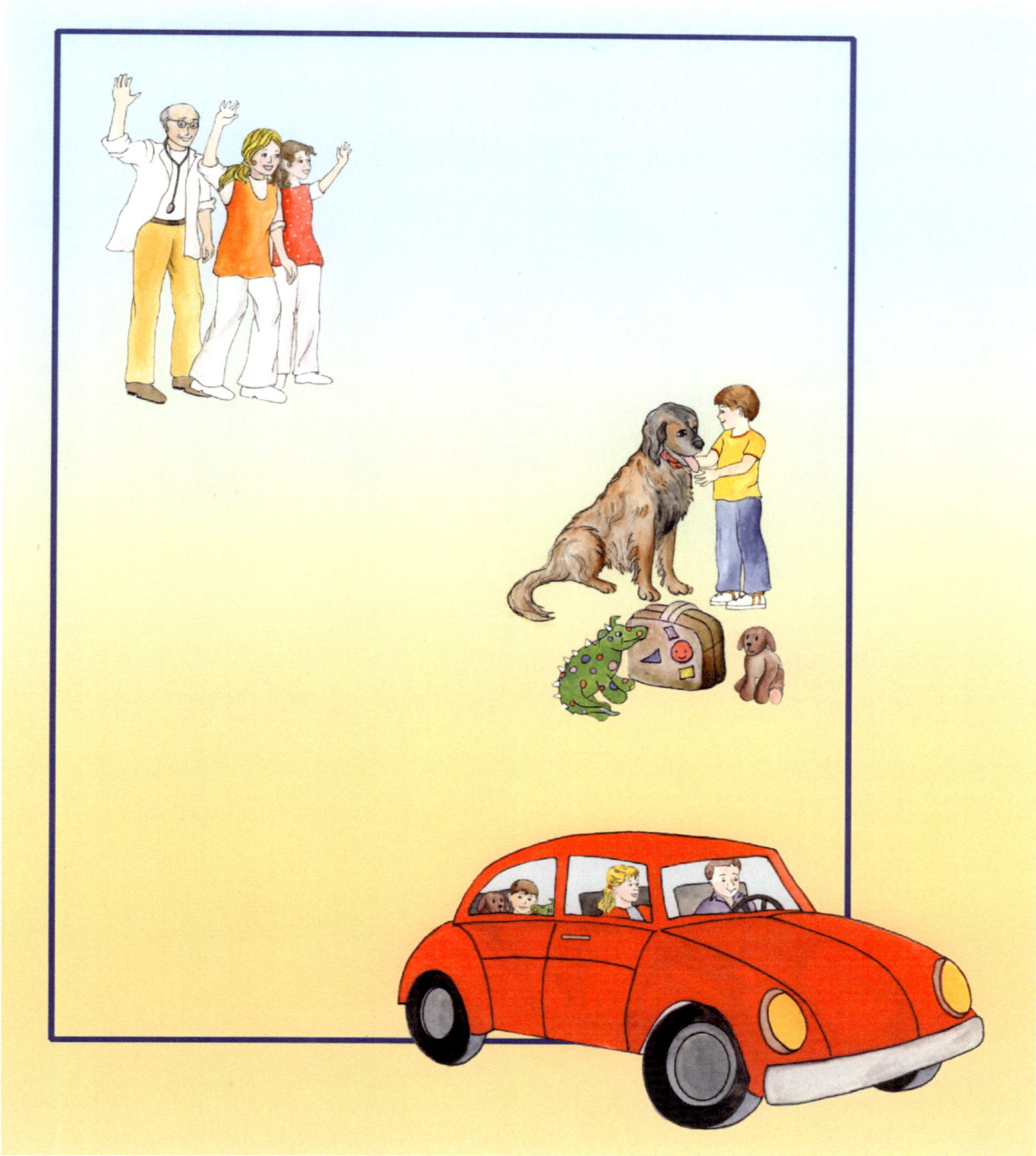

As Nurse Bobbi wheels Kirk through the big front door, Kirk gives high-fives to many of his new friends in the hospital. Nurse Bobbi helps him into the car, and Kirk waves good-bye to Rowan who is sitting in the doorway until the car disappears around the corner.

Rowan then happily trots back into the hospital, eager to meet other patients who will give her tummy rubs and big hugs.

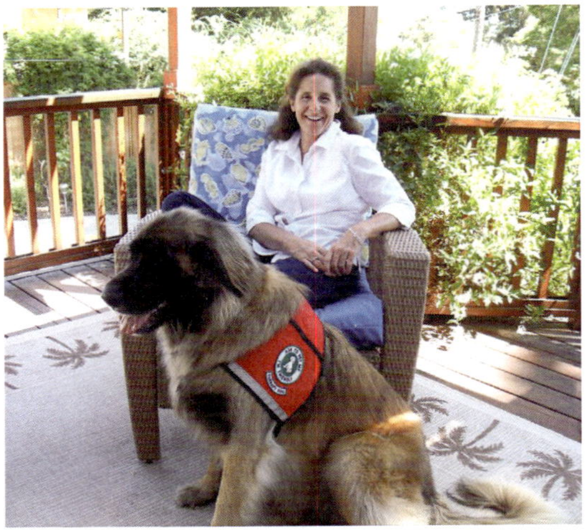

Jaynie Wood is a native of Santa Barbara, California where she lives and works. She is a Child Life Specialist with a Master's degree from the University of LaVerne and was instrumental in creating the Cottage Hospital CLS program, now in its 12th year. She enjoys spending time with her 3-year-old Leonberger, Rowan, a Pet Assisted Therapy Dog. In addition to her full-time position at Cottage, she and Rowan spend much of their time visiting pediatric patients in the hospital where Jaynie was born. She feels she has come full circle.

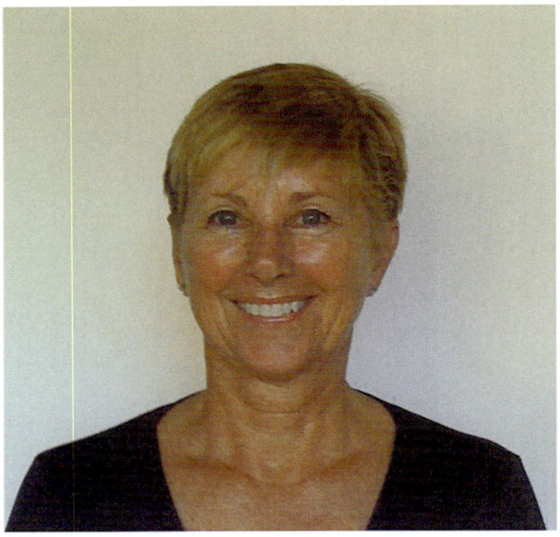

Jo Berkus is an English Major and an avid sports woman. She feels very blessed to have a blended family which includes eight remarkable grandchildren.

She served in the Special Olympics under Eunice Shriver and taught sports to children world-wide. She was twice the Women's World Champion in Frisbee and was the first woman inducted into the Frisbee Hall of Fame.

She currently serves on the Teddy Bear Cancer Foundation Board, and volunteers in the pediatric ward at Santa Barbara Cottage Hospital.

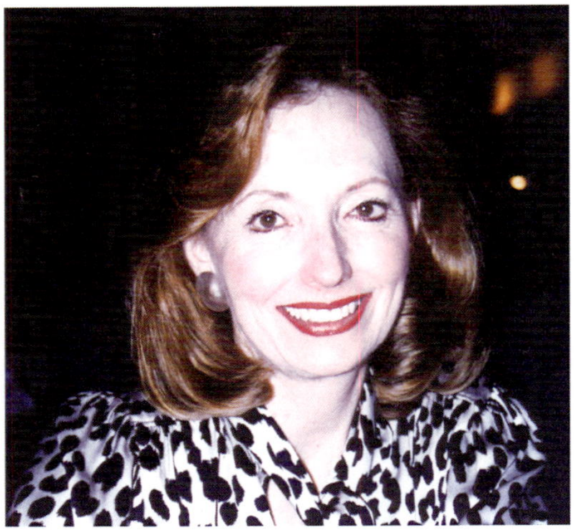

Joan Selwyn is an accomplished artist and illustrator. She taught art at the Los Angeles County Museum of Art, and is a collector of vintage children's books. She published her first book in 2002 (*ABC Dragons*) which she wrote and illustrated. She studied graphic design at UCLA and has utilized those skills for individuals, companies, and non-profits.

She is an educator, an art director and has served on the Boards of many institutions including the Board of the Otis Art Institute, Music Academy of the West, Blue Ribbon Los Angeles County Music Center and was Protocol Manager for the 1984 Olympic Art Festival.